The Tastiest Fat Bombs Recipes

Keto-Friendly Recipes That Will Satisfy Your Craving for Sweet

BY: Valeria Ray

License Notes

A Special Reward for Purchasing My Book!

Thank you, cherished reader, for purchasing my book and taking the time to read it. As a special reward for your decision, I would like to offer a gift of free and discounted books directly to your inbox. All you need to do is fill in the box below with your email address and name to start getting amazing offers in the comfort of your own home. You will never miss an offer because a reminder will be sent to you. Never miss a deal and get great deals without having to leave the house! Subscribe now and start saving!

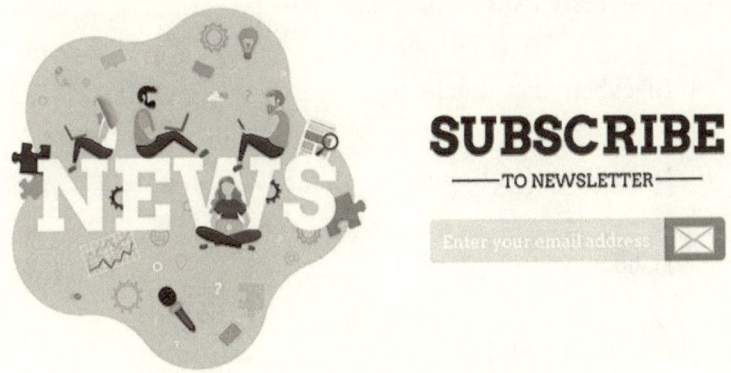

https://valeria-ray.gr8.com

Contents

Fat Bombs Recipes

MMMMMMMMMMMMMMMMMMMMMMMMMMMMMMMM

(1) Ginger Coconut Fat Bombs

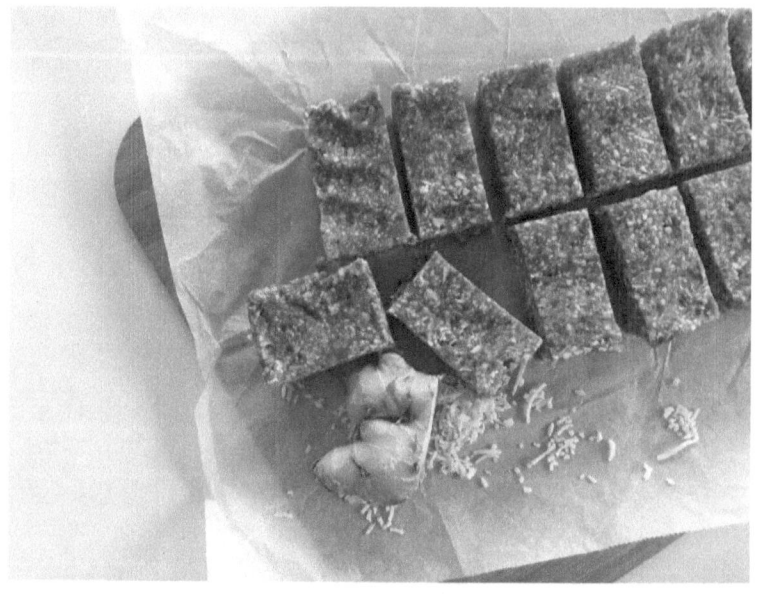

Ginger with coconut, doest sound delicious. This fat bomb recipe has brought them together with the sweet mix of coconut butter. Avoid using fresh or dried ginger, as only the powder can keep up the smooth consistency of the buttery blend.

Yield: 12

Prep Time: 10minutes

Cook Time: 0 minutes

List of Ingredients:

- 1 ¼ cup coconut butter softened
- 1 ¼ cup coconut oil softened
- 4 tbsp. shredded coconut unsweetened
- Sugar, to taste
- 2 tsp. ginger powder

MMMMMMMMMMMMMMMMMMMMMMMMMMMMMMMMMMM

Methods:

1. Blend all the ingredients in a blender.
2. Divide the mixture into the silicone molds.
3. Freeze for 10 minutes.
4. Serve.

(2) Mayo Salmon Bombs

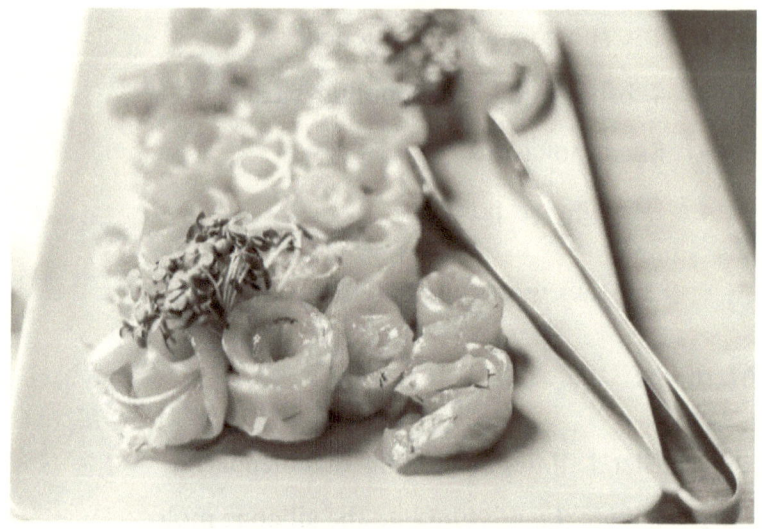

These colorful salmon balls are loved for their fine appeal and aroma. Salmon lover will enjoy them to the core. It has mayo mixed with salmon and chives. Addition of eggs makes them best suited for breakfast.

Yield: 08

Prep Time: 10 minutes

Cook Time: 0 minutes

List of Ingredients:

- 8 oz. smoked salmon, sliced
- 1 tbsp. butter, salted
- 4 large eggs
- 4 tbsp. fresh chives, chopped
- Salt and pepper to taste
- 4 tbsp. mayonnaise

MMMMMMMMMMMMMMMMMMMMMMMMMMMMMMMMMM

Methods:

1. Take a small cooking pot and fill it water. Bring the water to a boil.
2. Add two eggs to the water and let them fully boil for 12 minutes.
3. Heat 2 tsp. butter in a skillet and add salmon slices.
4. Sauté salmon until crispy then set it aside.
5. Peel eggs and place them in a bowl.
6. Mash these eggs with a fork.
7. Add half of the salmon and chives, mayonnaise, butter, salt, and pepper.
8. Mix well then make small balls using this mixture.
9. Mix remaining chives and salmon in a plate.
10. Roll the balls in the chive's mixture and coat well.
11. Serve.

(3) Granola Fat Bombs

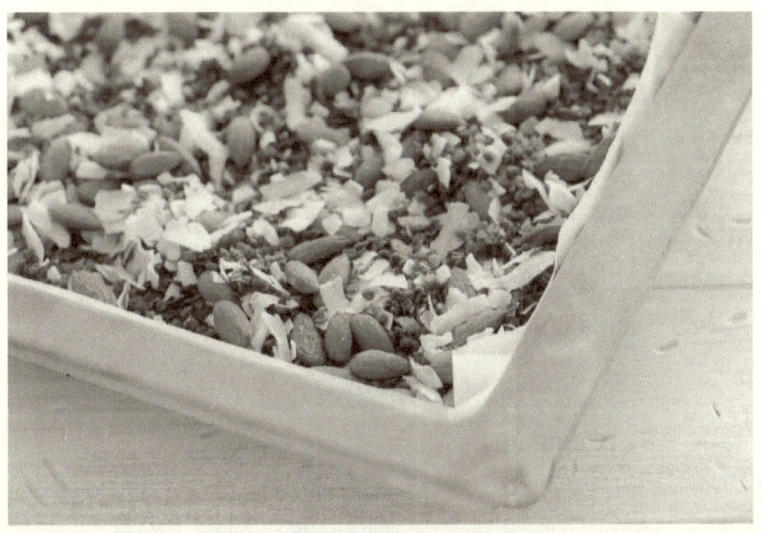

Granola is loved and tried in every possible variety.
Granola is basically any coarse mixture of substances. It
can either be sweet or salty. Here it is seasoned with pink
salt and delicious coconut shavings.

Yield: 12

Prep Time: 10minutes

Cook Time: 0 minutes

List of Ingredients:

- 7 oz sugar-free chocolate
- 2 cups Natural Peanut (or you can use Almond Butter)
- ½ cup of grass fed unsalted butter
- ½ cup coconut oil
- 1 cup of unsweetened coconut shavings
- 5 cups nuts & seeds
- ½ tsp. kosher or pink salt
- 1 tsp. cinnamon

MMMMMMMMMMMMMMMMMMMMMMMMMMMMMMM

Methods:

1. Layer 24 muffin cups with paper liners and set it aside.
2. Mix nut butter, chocolate, coconut oil, butter and syrup in a bowl.
3. Melt this mixture in the microwave for 30 seconds.
4. Stir well then fold in seeds, nuts, salt, cinnamon, and coconut shavings.
5. Mix well and divide the mixture into the lined muffin cups.
6. Refrigerate for 3 hours.
7. Remove the bombs from the muffin cups.
8. Serve.

(4) Green Mocha Fat Bomb

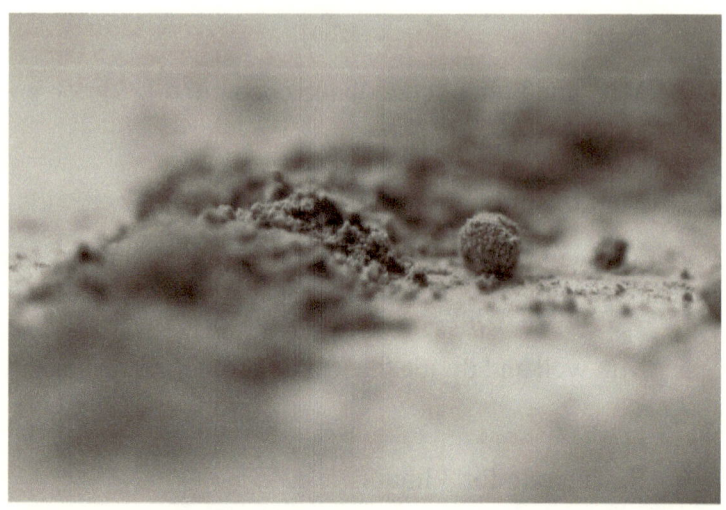

These mocha fat bombs are not only soothing for the site, but they also taste amazing. These are the perfect mix of avocados, Matcha powder, and cream. This is perhaps the most delicious way to add avocados to your diet. Try them, especially for kids.

Yield: 03

Prep Time: 10 minutes

Cook Time: 0minutes

List of Ingredients:

- 1 medium avocado
- 1 ½ scoops mct powder
- ½ tbsp. Matcha green tea powder (organic would be best)
- 1 tbsp. monk fruit sweetener
- ½ tsp. organic vanilla extract
- 1 ½ tbsp. coconut oil
- 1 tbsp. coconut cream

for the coating

- 1 tbsp. organic Matcha green tea powder
- 1 tbsp. of powdered monk fruit sweetener

MMMMMMMMMMMMMMMMMMMMMMMMMMMMMMMMMM

Methods:

1. Blend all the ingredients in a blender.
2. Refrigerate the mixture for 30 minutes.
3. Make about 12 small balls out of this mixture.
4. Mix coating ingredients in a shallows bowl.
5. Roll the balls in this mixture to coat well.
6. Serve.

(5) Cream Banana Fat Bombs

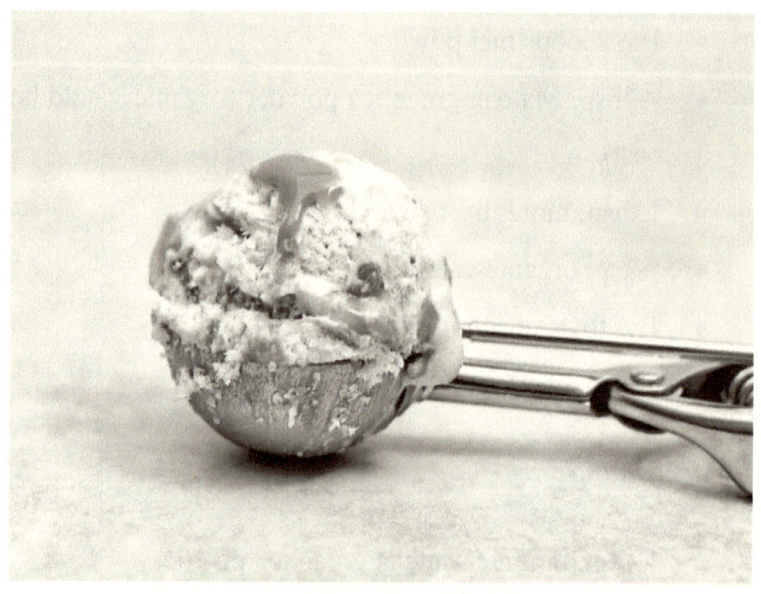

Add a twist to the plain cream cheese fats with some banana extract. Here you can also try some banana mash, but extract is best to keep the color of the bombs fresh and to get a creamy smooth texture.

Yield: 12

Prep Time: 10minutes

Cook Time: 0 minutes

List of Ingredients:

- 2 ½ cups cream cheese
- 1 ½ cup heavy whipping cream
- 2 tbsp. banana extract
- Stevia drops, to taste
- 2 tsp. Sugar

MMMMMMMMMMMMMMMMMMMMMMMMMMMMMMMMM

Methods:

1. Grease 30 silicone mold with cooking spray.
2. Beat heavy cream with cream cheese, banana extract, and sweeteners for 5 minutes.
3. Divide this mixture into the silicone molds.
4. Freeze the bombs for 1 hour.
5. Remove the bombs from the molds.
6. Serve.

(6) Bacon Egg Bombs

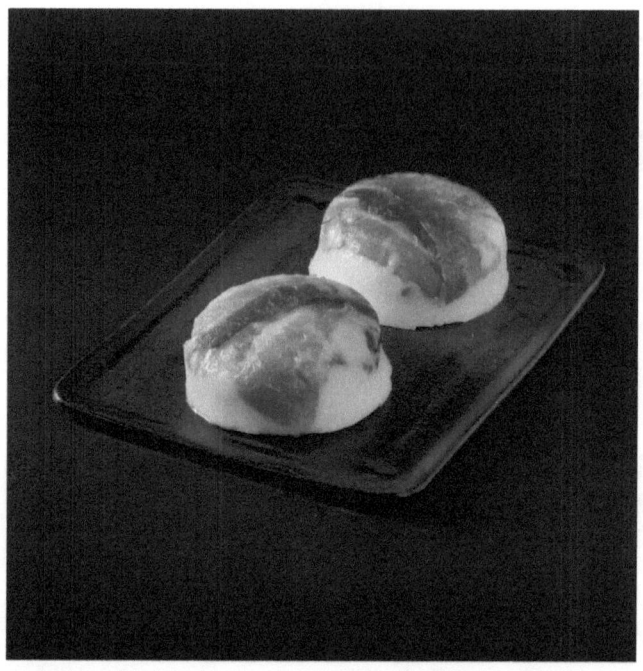

This bacon egg bomb is a good option for the morning meal. If you are bored with plain omelettes or boiled eggs, then try these. They are made out of egg, mayonnaise, and bacon in proportion. Eggs are mashed well and then seasoned with salt and pepper. You can preserve its make ahead in the refrigerator for about 2 days.

Yield: 12

Prep Time:5 minutes

Cook Time: 15 minutes

List of Ingredients:

- 2 large eggs
- ½ cup butter or ghee, softened
- 4 tbsp. mayonnaise
- freshly ground black pepper
- Salt to taste
- 8 large slices bacon

MMMMMMMMMMMMMMMMMMMMMMMMMMMMMMMMMM

Methods:

1. Set your oven to 375 degrees F. Layer a baking sheet with a parchment paper.
2. Place the bacon strips in the baking sheet in a single layer and bake for 15 minutes.
3. Boil all the eggs in a saucepan filled with water.
4. Once the eggs are hard-boiled transfer them to an ice bath, then peel.
5. Add peeled egg to a bowl along with butter and mash well with a fork.
6. Stir in salt, pepper, and mayonnaise. Mix well then pour in baked bacon grease.
7. Mix well and refrigerate for 30 minutes.
8. Crumble the baked bacon in a plate.
9. Make 6 small balls out of the refrigerated eggs mixture.
10. Roll these balls in the crumbled bacon.
11. Serve and enjoy.

(7) Strawberry Fat Bombs

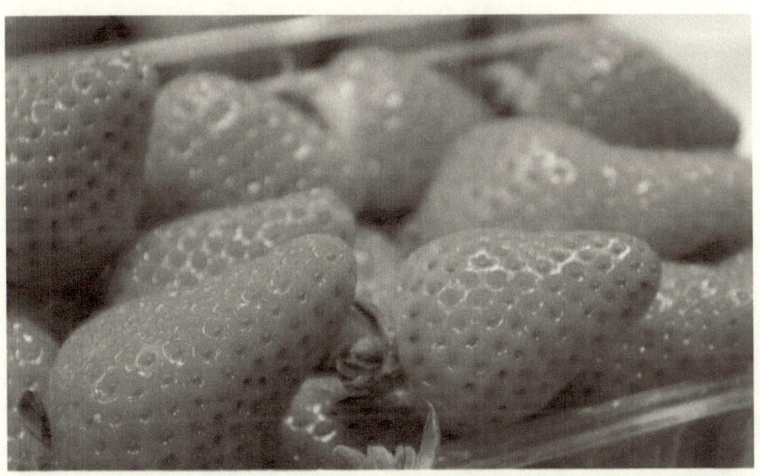

How can we forget the delectable strawberry flavor? These fat bombs are all about strawberries. The juicy blend of the berries is mixed with coconut shred and butter. Serve with a refreshing strawberry smoothie to experience the best of its flavor.

Yield: 12

Prep Time: 10minutes

Cook Time: 0 minutes

List of Ingredients:

- 1 ½ cup almond flour
- ½ cup coconut flour
- ½ cup shredded coconut
- 1 cup strawberries
- 2 tsp. vanilla extract
- 2 tbsp. coconut oil
- 2 tsp. stevia

MMMMMMMMMMMMMMMMMMMMMMMMMMMMMMMMM

Methods:

1. Blend all the ingredients except coconut shreds in a food processor.
2. Use this mixture to make small bite-sized balls.
3. Roll these balls in the shredded coconut.
4. Freeze the balls for 1 hour.
5. Serve.

(8) Blackberry Fat Bombs

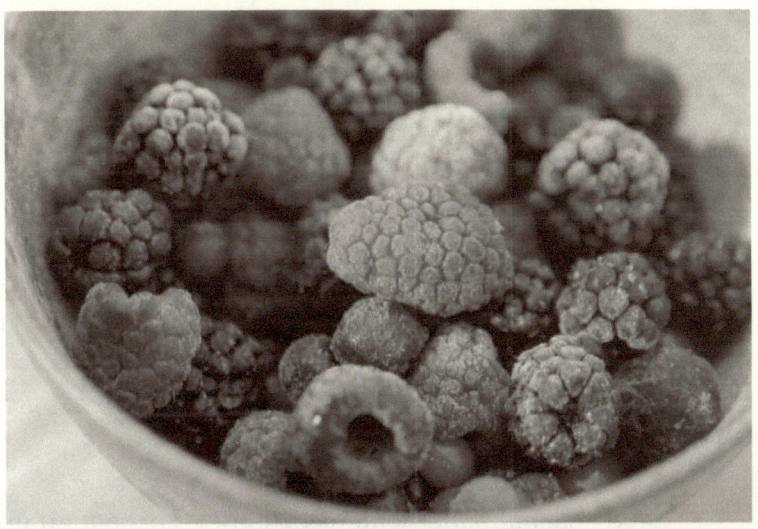

As fascinating as these fat bombs look, they taste delicious.
Blackberries lover will instantly fall for these .They have a
mildly sweet taste with an infused flavors of vanilla along
with some lemon juice. You can switch coconut butter with
any other butter of your choice.

Yield: 3

Prep Time: 15 minutes

Cook Time: 0 minutes

List of Ingredients:

- ½ cup coconut butter
- ½ cup coconut oil
- ¼ cup fresh or frozen blackberries
- 2 tsp. honey
- 1/8 tsp. vanilla powder
- ½ tbsp. lemon juice

MMMMMMMMMMMMMMMMMMMMMMMMMMMMMMMMM

Methods:

1. Add coconut butter with blackberries, coconut oil in a cooking pot.
2. Cook until all the ingredients are mixed.
3. Transfer the mixture to a blender with all the remaining ingredients.
4. Blend well until smooth.
5. Line a 6-inch pan with parchment paper.
6. Pour the blackberry mixture into the pan and spread it evenly.
7. Refrigerate it for one hour.
8. Remove the pan and slice the bar into small squares.
9. Serve.

(9) Mixed Nuts Fat Bombs

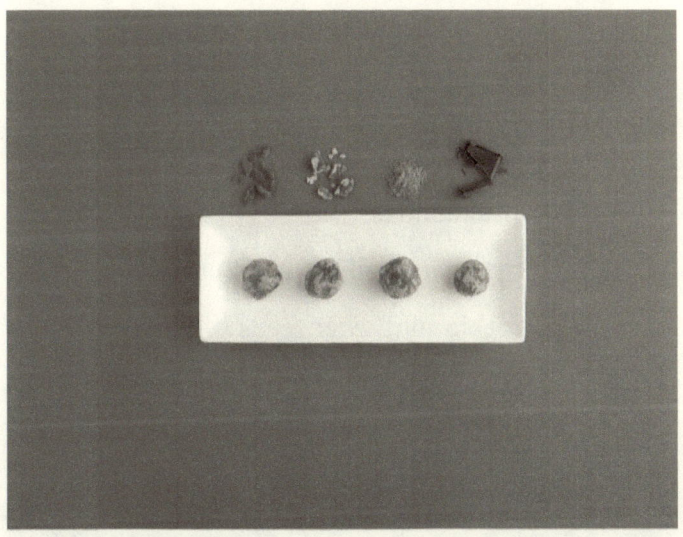

Another good addition to the Matcha series of fat bombs. These unique in texture, color, and taste. With the added cashews, flower seeds, pumpkin seeds and almonds, the blend is a complete package in its self.

Yield: 12

Prep Time: 10minutes

Cook Time: 0 minutes

List of Ingredients:

- 1 cup coconut oil
- ½ cup coconut butter
- 2 cups organic shredded coconut
- 1 cup raw cashew
- 1 cup raw almonds
- ½ cup organic unshelled pumpkin seeds
- ½ cup organic sunflower seeds
- 2/3 cup unsweetened vanilla almond milk
- 2 tsp. cinnamon
- 4 tsp. Matcha powder

MMMMMMMMMMMMMMMMMMMMMMMMMMMMMMMMM

Methods:

1. Blend all the ingredients in a blender.
2. Use this mixture to make 1-inch small balls.
3. Arrange the balls in a tray lined with parchment paper.
4. Freeze for 1 hour.
5. Serve.

(10) Chocolate Chip Fat Bombs

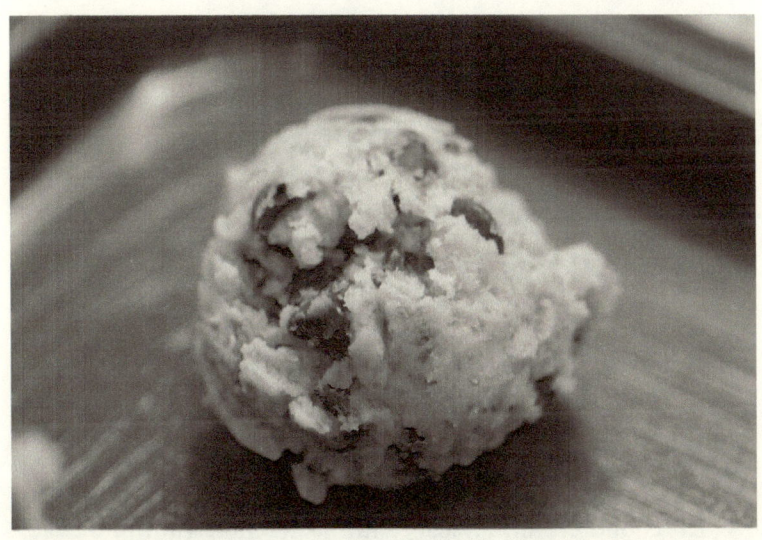

These cream cheese chocolate chip fat bombs are best for desserts. When served well chilled on a warm summer day, you will love them. You can store the cream cheese make ahead in the refrigerator for as many as 2 to 3 days.

Yield: 3

Prep Time: 10minutes

Cook Time: 0 minutes

List of Ingredients:

- 2 oz. cream cheese softened
- 2 tbsp. melted butter
- 2 tbsp. coconut oil
- 1 tbsp. sugar
- 2 tbsp. sugar-free chocolate chips
- ½ tsp. vanilla extract

MMMMMMMMMMMMMMMMMMMMMMMMMMMMMMMMMM

Methods:

1. Blend cream cheese with sweetener, vanilla extract, coconut oil and melted butter in a blender.
2. Fold in chocolate chips and mix gently.
3. Line a muffin tray with parchment liners.
4. Divide the cream cheese mixture into the muffin cups.
5. Freeze for 30 minutes.
6. Serve

(11) Cheesy Egg Bombs

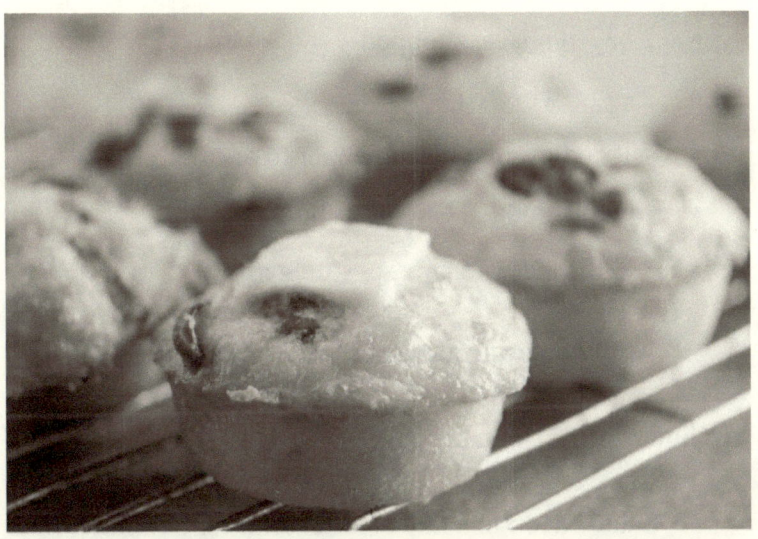

Here is another good breakfast option to try for an energized morning. Besides eggs and bacon, these fat bombs also carry cream cheese and shredded cheddar, leaving them more enriched and nutritious.

Yield: 2

Prep Time: 05 minutes

Cook Time: 10 minutes

List of Ingredients:

- 1 tbsp. butter, divided
- 2 bacon slices, chopped
- 2 eggs, whisked
- salt and ground black pepper to taste
- ¾ cup shredded Cheddar cheese
- 2 ½ tbsp. cream cheese, softened

MMMMMMMMMMMMMMMMMMMMMMMMMMMMMMMMMM

Methods:

1. Sauté bacon in a large skillet until for 8 minutes then transfer to a plate lined with paper towel.
2. Set your oven to 400 degrees F. Oil a 9-inch pie plate.
3. Melt butter in a skillet and add eggs. Stir cook for 5 minutes.
4. Adjust seasoning with salt and pepper.
5. Mix scrambled eggs with shredded cheese.
6. Make small balls out of this mixture.
7. Crumble sautéed bacon in a plate.
8. Roll the balls in the bacon.
9. Serve.

(12) Chocolate Fat Bombs

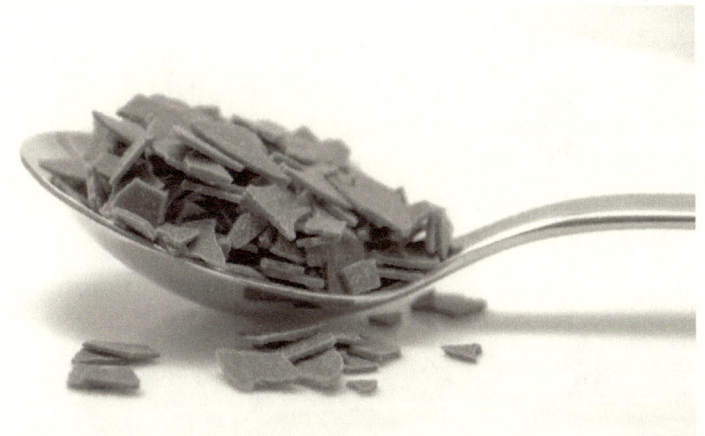

Best for simple desserts, these chocolate fat bombs are a peanut butter variety with easy to set and store texture. For good result at least refrigerate the chocolate mixture for a 1 hour, else they won't turn as firm.

Yield: 6

Prep Time: 10minutes

Cook Time: 0 minutes

List of Ingredients:

- ½ cup no sugar peanut butter
- ½ cup coconut oil
- 2-oz. unsweetened baking chocolate
- 2 tbsp. cocoa
- 1 tsp. vanilla stevia drops

MMMMMMMMMMMMMMMMMMMMMMMMMMMMMMMMM

Methods:

1. Mix melted peanut butter, baking chocolate, cocoa and coconut oil in a bowl.
2. Stir in stevia and mix well until combined.
3. Divide this mixture into the silicone molds.
4. Freeze for 1 hour.
5. Remove the bombs from the molds.
6. Serve.

(13) Jalapeño Gruyere Fat Bombs

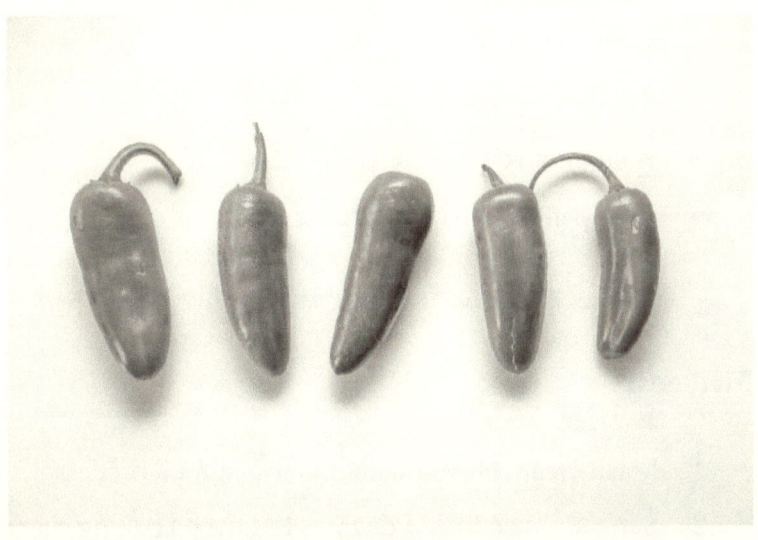

You may have already tried the good old jalapeno poppers; these fat bombs will bring you the same distinct jalapeno flavor with the added richness of the gruyere cheese. Cream cheese is added to give a thick creamy base to the balls, and the bacon is there to coat them in extra crispiness.

Yield: 12

Prep Time: 10 minutes

Cook Time: 30 minutes

List of Ingredients:

- 7 oz. full-fat cream cheese
- ½ cup unsalted butter
- 8 slices no sugar bacon
- ½ cup grated Gruyere cheese
- 4 jalapeño peppers halved, seeded

MMMMMMMMMMMMMMMMMMMMMMMMMMMMMMMMMMM

Methods:

1. Mash cream cheese with butter in a food processor.
2. Set your oven to 325 degrees F. Layer a baking sheet with parchment paper.
3. Place the bacon strips in the baking sheet in a single layer and bake for 30 minutes.
4. Allow the bacon to cool then crumble it in a plate. Set it aside.
5. Add jalapeno, bacon grease and cheese to the cream cheese mixture.
6. Mix well and refrigerate for 30 minutes.
7. Make 6 balls out of this refrigerated mixture.
8. Roll them in the crumbled bacon.
9. Serve.

(14) Peanut Butter Protein Bombs

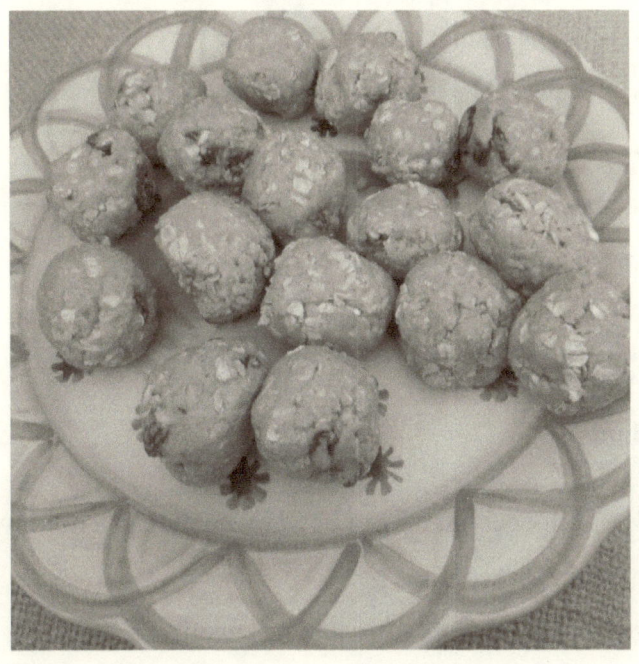

Yield: 12

Prep Time: 10minutes

Cook Time: 2 minutes

List of Ingredients:

- 2 cups coconut oil
- 2 cups peanut butter
- 1 cup cocoa powder
- ½ cup plant-based protein powder
- 2 pinches of sea salt
- Unsweetened shredded coconut

MMMMMMMMMMMMMMMMMMMMMMMMMMMMMMMMM

Methods:

1. Melt coconut oil in a bowl by heating in a microwave for 30 seconds.
2. Stir in peanut butter and mix well.
3. Add protein powder, salt, and cocoa powder. Mix well to combine.
4. Prepare small balls out of this mixture and arrange them on a tray.
5. Freeze this mixture for 15 minutes.
6. Place coconut shred in a plate.
7. Roll the frozen fat bombs in the coconut shreds to coat.
8. Serve.

(15) Cream Cheese Matcha Bombs

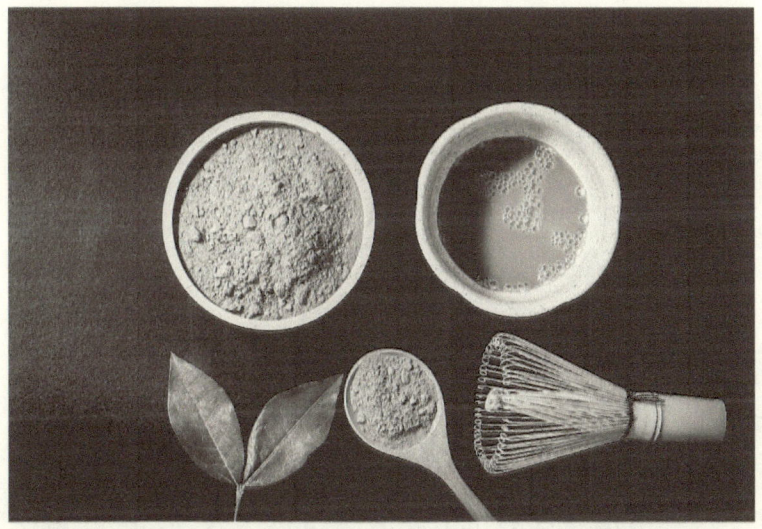

These green fat bombs are all Matcha, mixed with cream cheese and cinnamon. These spices are adding a strong and sharp flavor to the bombs. These fat bombs are best to serve as evening or party snacks. Use any mold of your choice to get the desired shapes.

Yield: 12

Prep Time: 10 minutes

Cook Time: 1 minute

List of Ingredients:

- 1 cup raw cocoa butter
- 2 tbsp. coconut oil
- 2 tbsp. cream cheese, softened
- 2 scoop Matcha MCT Oil Powder
- 1 tsp. cinnamon
- ½ cup HWC

MMMMMMMMMMMMMMMMMMMMMMMMMMMMMMM

Methods:

1. Melt cocoa butter in a bowl by heating in a microwave for 30 seconds.
2. Blend all the ingredients including melted butter in a bowl using an electric mixer.
3. Pour this mixture into silicone molds and freeze for 4 hours immediately.
4. Remove the bombs from the molds and serve.

(16) Blueberry Lemon Fat Bombs

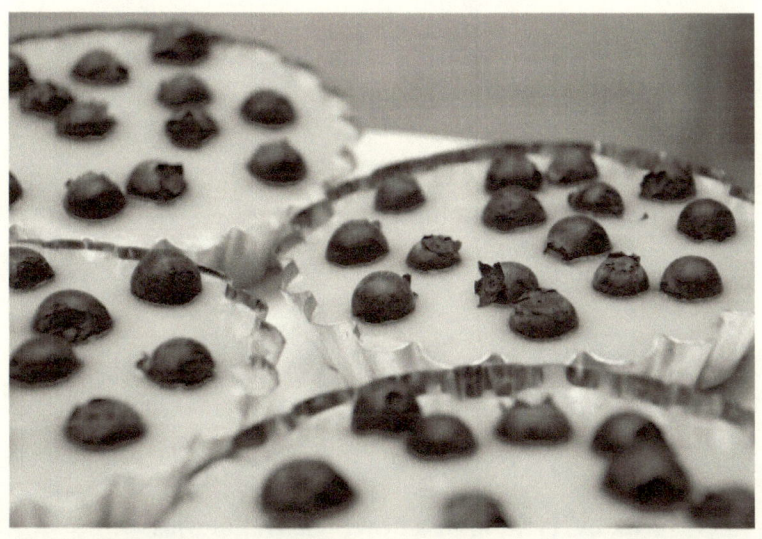

These black eyes fats bombs are actually lemon based blueberry fat bombs. Due to their mild taste and appealing presentation you can serve these at all sorts of festive occasions. Try to use fresh berries for more inspiring flavor.

Yield: 12

Prep Time: 10minutes

Cook Time: 0 minutes

List of Ingredients:

- 1 cup coconut oil, melted
- 2 tbsp. lemon zest the
- 6 tbsp. lemon juice
- Sugar , to taste
- 1 ½ cup coconut butter
- 32 blueberries

MMMMMMMMMMMMMMMMMMMMMMMMMMMMMMMMMMM

Methods:

1. Mix everything in a bowl without berries.
2. Place 1 berry at the bottom of silicon molds.
3. Divide the lemon mixture into the silicone mold.
4. Refrigerate for 30 minutes to 1 hour.
5. Serve.

(17) Coco Coconut Bombs

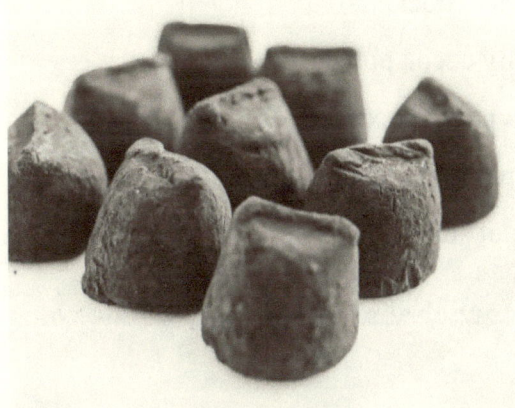

Chocolate is all time favorite of everybody. These choco bombs will bring extra pleasure to the chocolate lovers as they are loaded with cocoa powder and a coconut shreds. Milk and butter are used to give the base. However you can also use cream to enjoy some extra richness.

Yield: 3

Prep Time: 10 minutes

Cook Time: 5 minutes

List of Ingredients:

- ½ cup coconut butter
- ½ cup coconut milk
- ½ tsp. vanilla extract
- 2 tbsp. quality cocoa powder
- ½ tsp. stevia powder extract
- 2 drops peppermint essential oil
- ½ cup coconut shreds

MMMMMMMMMMMMMMMMMMMMMMMMMMMMMMMMM

Methods:

1. Heat water in a large saucepan and place a glass bowl in it.
2. Add all the ingredients to the bowl except coconut shred.
3. Cook until all the ingredients melt together in the bowl. Mix well.
4. Remove the bowl from the pan and refrigerate for 30 minutes.
5. Make small 1-inch balls out this refrigerated mixture.
6. Roll the balls in the coconut shreds to coat well.
7. Refrigerate for 1 hour.
8. Serve.

(18) Vanilla Nut Fat Bombs

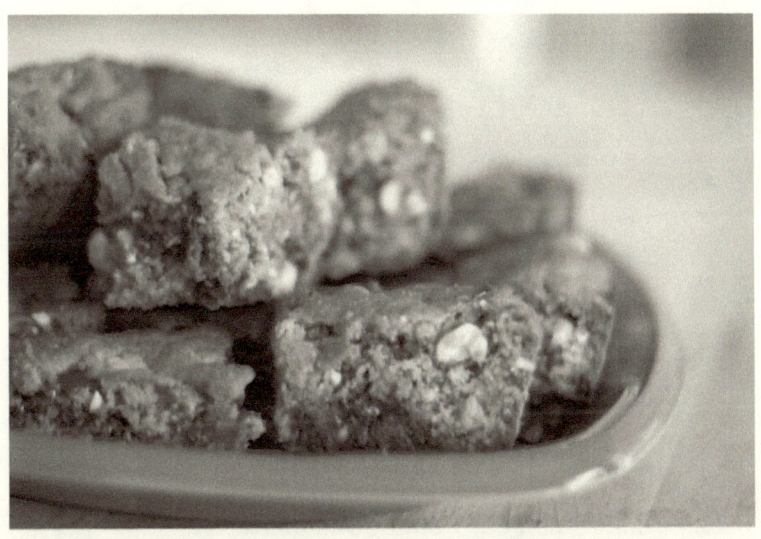

Let's try something nuttier. These fats bombs are made out of a rich, crunchy mix of nuts. Here you have a complete choice to add your favorite nuts, try either almonds or pecan or walnuts or a combination of all these.

Yield: 12

Prep Time: 10minutes

Cook Time: 0 minutes

List of Ingredients:

- ½ cup coconut oil
- 2 cups nuts of your choice
- ½ cup butter
- 4 tsp. vanilla extract
- Sugar , to taste

MMMMMMMMMMMMMMMMMMMMMMMMMMMMMMMMMM

Methods:

1. Blend all the ingredients in a blender.
2. Make small balls out of this mixture.
3. Freeze for about 1 hour.
4. Serve.

(19) Bacon Avocado Fat Bombs

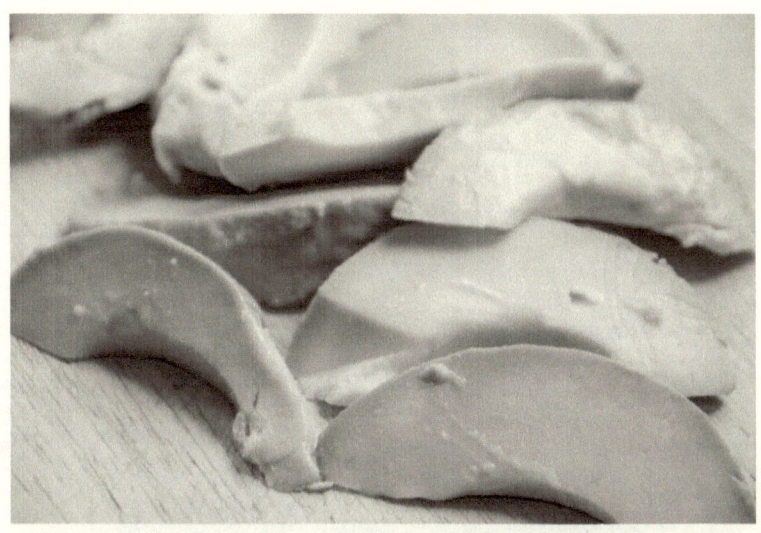

Bringing all your favorite breakfast meals together into one, these fats bombs are an amazing mix of avocado with bacon. Onion, chili pepper, and butter are mixed well to create a crunchy and juicy flavor in each bite. Mashed avocado flesh is serving as an excellent base for the bombs.

Yield: 3

Prep Time: 5 minutes

Cook Time: 15 minutes

List of Ingredients:

- 2 slices bacon
- ½ small avocado
- ½ tbsp. fresh lime juice
- 2 tbsp. butter
- ½ tbsp. onion diced
- ½ cloves garlic crushed
- ½ tbsp. cilantro chopped
- ½ small chili pepper finely chopped
- salt and pepper to taste

MMMMMMMMMMMMMMMMMMMMMMMMMMMMMMMM

Methods:

1. Set your oven to 375 degrees F. Layer a baking sheet with a parchment paper.
2. Place the bacon strips in the baking sheet in a single layer and bake for 15 minutes.
3. Boil all the eggs in a saucepan filled with water.
4. Once the eggs are hard-boiled transfer them to an ice bath, then peel.
5. Add peeled egg to a bowl along with butter and mash well with a fork.
6. Stir in avocado flesh and mash again until well mixed.
7. Add all the remaining ingredients except bacon.
8. Mix well and refrigerate for 30 minutes.
9. Crumble the baked bacon in a plate.
10. Make 6 small balls out of the refrigerated eggs mixture.
11. Roll these balls in the crumbled bacon.
12. Serve and enjoy.

(20) Espresso Fat Bombs

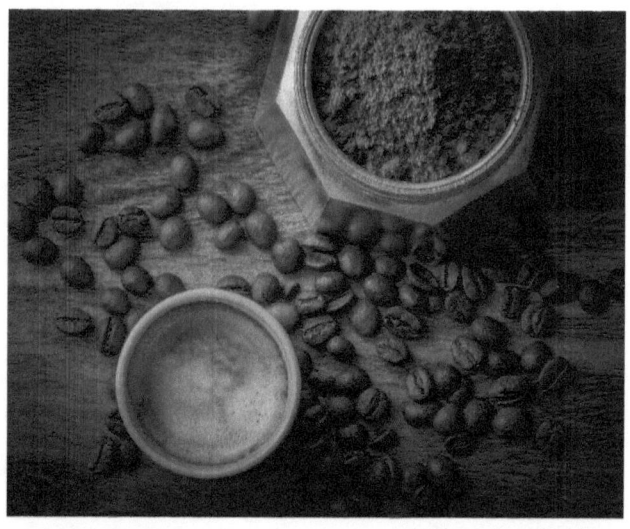

These espresso fat bombs are great for a kicking start in the morning. Or you can also serve them after a meal as a dessert. Since they are so high in calories and energy, keep theirs to a moderate level.

Yield: **12**

Prep Time: 10minutes

Cook Time: 0 minutes

List of Ingredients:

- 2/3 cup cashew or almond butter
- 2/3 cup coconut oil
- 3 tbsp. cacao powder
- 2 tbsp. coconut milk
- 3 tbsp. instant espresso powder
- Sugar , to taste

MMMMMMMMMMMMMMMMMMMMMMMMMMMMMMMM

Methods:

1. Combine all the ingredients over medium-low heat in a saucepan.
2. Stir in vanilla and salt. Mix well.
3. Divide this mixture into the silicone molds.
4. Freeze the bombs for 20 minutes.
5. Serve.

(21) Crunchy Cashew Fat Bombs

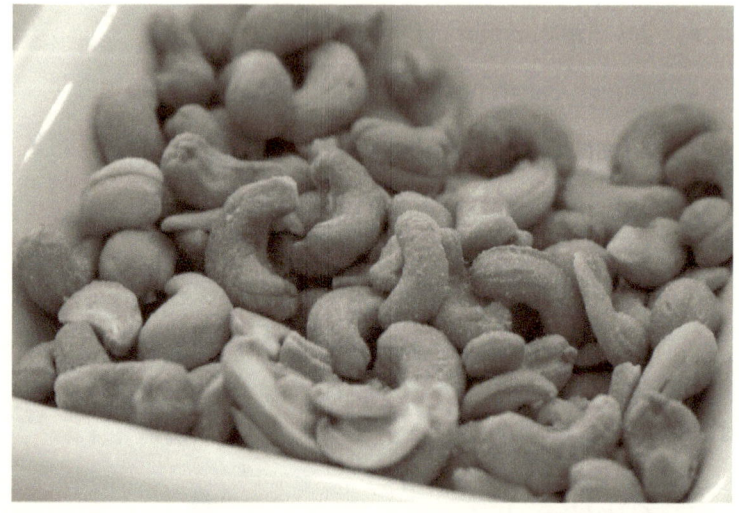

You are about to enjoy a deal full of crunch and crisp with these cashew fat bombs. Made out of butter and cocoa powder, these bombs are a delight to serve as after meal dessert or to serve with a cup of warm tea.

Yield: 08

Prep Time: 10 minutes

Cook Time: 1 minute

List of Ingredients:

- 2 cups Coconut Oil
- 2 cups Almond Butter
- ½ cup Coconut Flour
- 1 cup Cacao Powder
- 2 cups Raw Cashews

MMMMMMMMMMMMMMMMMMMMMMMMMMMMMMMMMM

Methods:

1. Heat coconut oil in a saucepan with almond butter. Mix well.
2. Mix coconut flour with cocoa powder in a bowl.
3. Stir in butter mixture and mix well to combine.
4. Refrigerate for 15 minutes.
5. Meanwhile, coarsely chop the cashews in a food processor.
6. Place the cashews in a plate and set it aside.
7. Take the coconut flour mixture and make small balls out of it.
8. Roll these balls in the chopped cashews.
9. Refrigerate for 5 minutes then enjoy.

(22) Raspberry Lime Fat Bombs

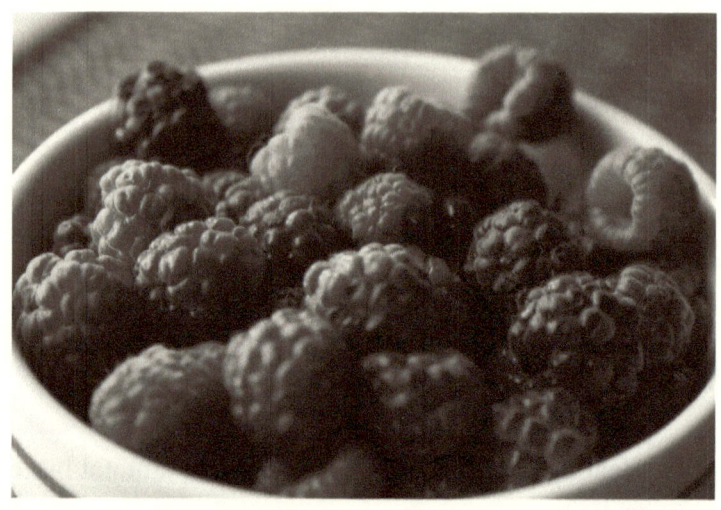

Imagining such a combination already takes us to the world of refreshing aromas and flavors. Make this real with this simple recipe of fresh raspberry fat bombs. Add lime juice for a refreshing twist.

Yield: 12

Prep Time: 10minutes

Cook Time: 1 minute

List of Ingredients:

- ½ cup melted coconut oil
- 8 tbsp. unsalted butter
- 8 oz. cream cheese
- Zest of 2 limes
- Juice of 1 lime
- Sugar , to taste
- ½ cup fresh raspberries

MMMMMMMMMMMMMMMMMMMMMMMMMMMMMMMMMMMM

Methods:

1. Heat coconut oil with cream cheese in the microwave for 30 seconds to melt.
2. Mix well until creamy.
3. Whisk in coconut oil, lime juice, sugar, and lime zest. Mix well.
4. Fold in fresh raspberries and mash them slightly with a fork.
5. Divide the mixture in the 16 silicon molds or do it in two batches of 8 molds.
6. Freeze for 2 hours.
7. Remove the bombs from the molds.
8. Serve.

(23) Creamy Blueberry Fat Bombs

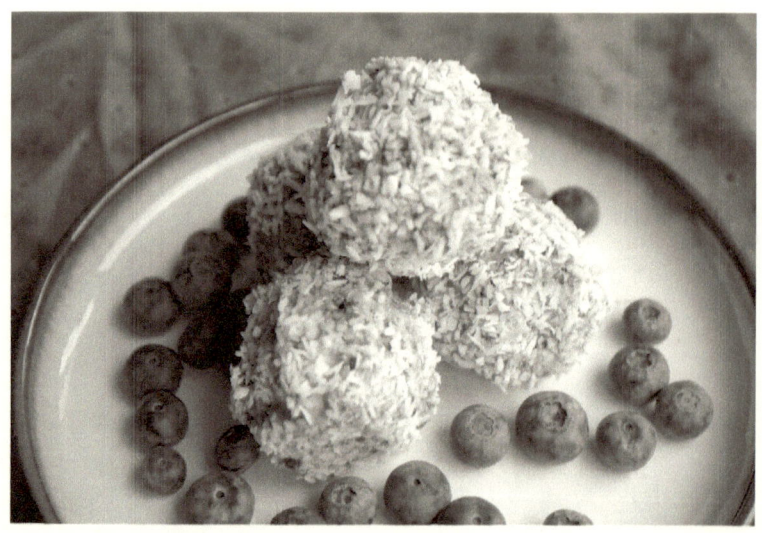

We all love blueberries, and these fat bombs capture the essence of fine berries into small crunchy bites. These bombs are based with blueberry mash, and then they are coated with coconut shreds.

Yield: 30

Prep Time: 10minutes

Cook Time: 0 minutes

List of Ingredients:

- 8 oz. soft goat cheese
- 1 cup fresh blueberries
- 2 cups almond flour
- 2 tsp. vanilla extract
- 1 cup pecans
- Sugar, to taste
- ½ cup unsweetened shredded coconut

MMMMMMMMMMMMMMMMMMMMMMMMMMMMMMMMMMMM

Methods:

1. Blend all the ingredients in a blender.
2. Make about 30 small balls out of this mixture.
3. Roll all the balls in the coconut flakes to coat well.
4. Serve.

(24) White Pecan Fat Bombs

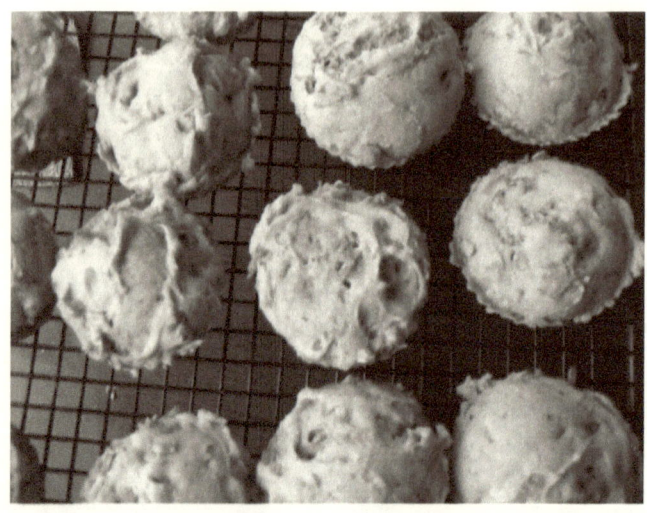

Enough with the dark chocolate, try something new and earthy with these white pecan fat bombs. These are made out of white chocolate blend, mixed with crunchy pecans. Use a variety of molds to get exciting shapes and sizes.

Prep Time: 10minutes

Cook Time: 2 minutes

Yield: 12

List of Ingredients:

- 4 tbsp. coconut oil
- 4 tbsp. butter
- 4 oz cocoa butter
- 4 tbsp. powdered sugar
- ½ tsp. vanilla extract
- 2 pinch brown sugar
- 2 pinch salt
- 1 cup chopped pecans

MMMMMMMMMMMMMMMMMMMMMMMMMMMMMMMMM

Methods:

1. Melt cocoa butter with butter and coconut oil in a small saucepan.
2. Blend this melted mixture with erythritol, vanilla extract and a pinch of salt.
3. Divide chopped pecans in the silicon molds.
4. Top the pecans with cocoa butter mixture in the molds.
5. Freeze for 30 minutes.
6. Serve.

(25) Tri-Layer Fat Bombs

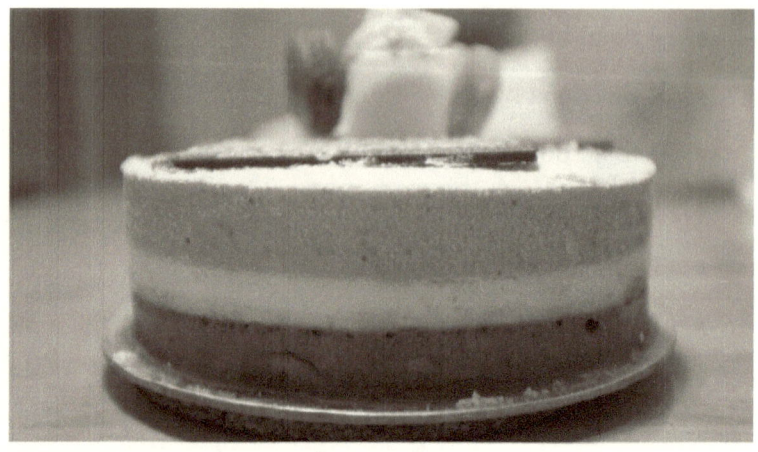

So many flavors in one bite! Kids will love you for these multi-layered fat bombs. A good blend of chocolate, strawberry, and vanilla is used in these frozen bites. Serve the bombs immediately after removing them from the molds.

Yield: 4

Prep Time: 10minutes

Cook Time: 0 minutes

List of Ingredients:

- ¼ cup butter
- ¼ cup coconut oil
- ¼ cup sour cream
- ¼ cup cream cheese
- 1 tbsp. brown sugar
- Honey, to taste
- 1 tbsp. cocoa powder
- ½ tsp. vanilla extract
- 1 medium strawberry

MMMMMMMMMMMMMMMMMMMMMMMMMMMMMMMM

Methods:

1. Mix coconut oil with butter, cream cheese, brown sugar, honey and sour cream in a bowl.
2. Blend all the ingredients in a blender.
3. Divide the mixture into 3 separate glass bowls.
4. Add cocoa powder to one bowl and mix well.
5. Strawberries to another bowl and vanilla to the third one.
6. Mix all the mixtures well then pour into separate silicon molds.
7. Freeze the fat bombs for 30 minutes.
8. Remove from the molds and serve.

(26) Creamy Peach Fat Bombs

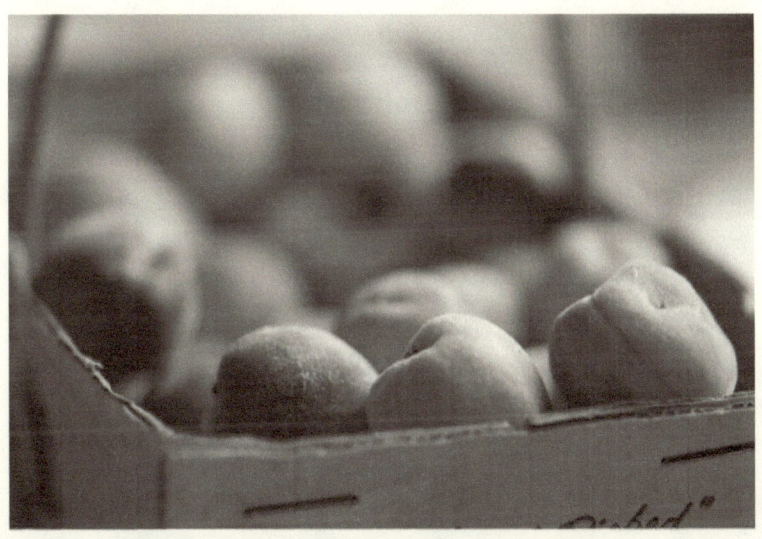

Add a refreshing touch to the creamy mascarpone fat bombs by adding peach extracts. Serve these with fresh peach slices and dive into new realms of taste. This super juicy treat is best for summer parties or evening snacks.

Yield: 12

Prep Time: 10minutes

Cook Time: 0 minutes

List of Ingredients:

- 2 oz. cream cheese softened
- 4 tbsp. butter, softened
- 8 oz., mascarpone, softened
- 4 tbsp. heavy whipping cream
- ½ cup sugar
- ½ tsp. vanilla extract
- ¼ tsp. peach extract
- 4 oz. weight fresh peaches, fine diced

MMMMMMMMMMMMMMMMMMMMMMMMMMMMMMMMMM

Methods:

1. Arrange 12 silicone molds in a cookie sheet and set it aside.
2. Blend mascarpone with butter, cream cheese in a blender.
3. Stir in peach extract, sweetener, and vanilla. Mix well.
4. Divide the mixture into the silicone molds.
5. Freeze for about 2 hours.
6. Serve.

(27) Double Layer Cheesecake Bombs

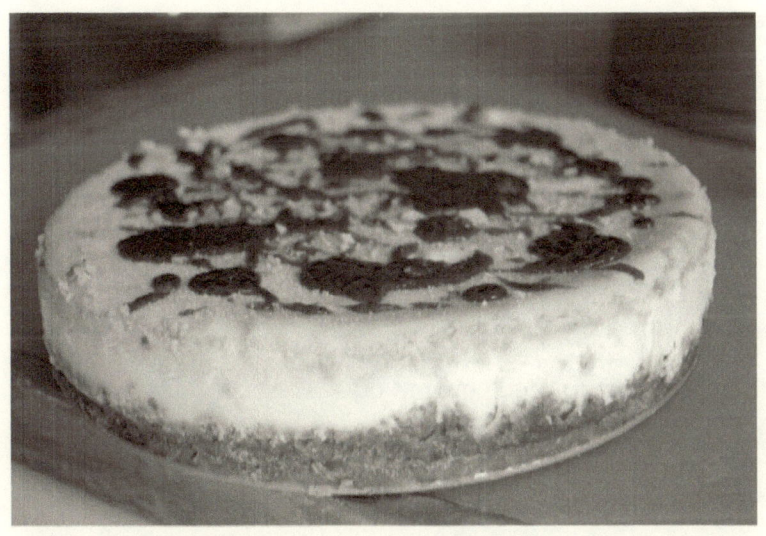

Now you can enjoy the cheesecake flavor fat bombs at home with a few simple ingredients and easy steps. This recipe is a double layered package which contains cheesecake layer the base and chocolate mixed layer on top.

Yield: 12

Prep Time: 10minutes

Cook Time: 0 minutes

List of Ingredients:

Base

- 2 cups cream cheese
- 4 tbsp. butter melted
- 2 tbsp. natvia (or erythritol)
- 2 tsp. vanilla extract
- ½ cups refined coconut oil

top

- 1 cup refined coconut oil
- 2 tsp. cocoa powder
- 4 tsp. natvia (or erythritol)

MMMMMMMMMMMMMMMMMMMMMMMMMMMMMMMM

Methods:

1. Blend butter with cream cheese in an electric mixer.
2. Stir in natvia, coconut oil, and vanilla. Blend well.
3. Divide the mixture into the silicone molds.
4. Freeze for about 20 minutes.
5. Mix coconut oil with natvia and cocoa powder in a bowl.
6. Pour this mixture over the frozen fat bombs.
7. Serve.

(28) Chocolate Cherry Fat Bombs

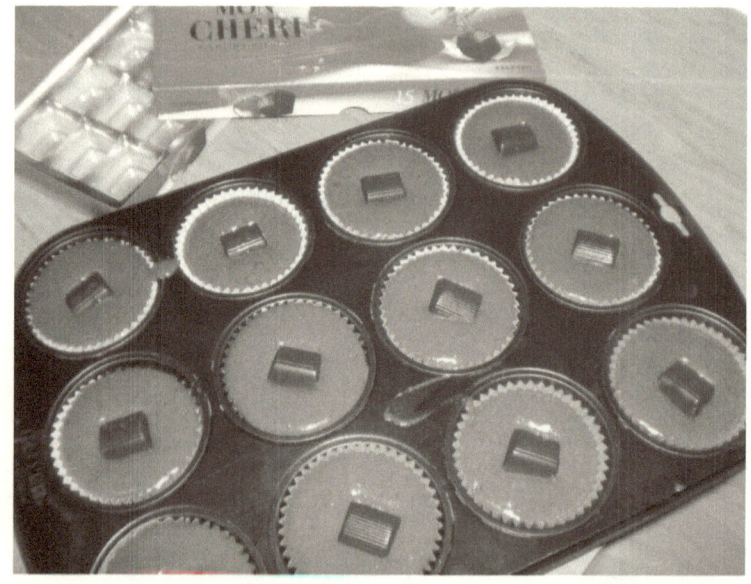

Surprise everyone with this one of a kind chocolate fat bombs, stuffed with a cherry on the inside. Dark thawed cherries are mixed with the chocolate rich blend and then frozen into these delicious bites.

Yield: 12

Prep Time: 10minutes

Cook Time: 0 minutes

List of Ingredients:

- 1 tsp. almond extract
- ½ cup coconut butter
- Sugar , to taste
- ½ cup coconut oil
- 1 ½ cup frozen dark cherries thawed
- 1 tsp. vanilla extract
- 6 tbsp. cacao powder

MMMMMMMMMMMMMMMMMMMMMMMMMMMMMMMMMM

Methods:

1. Whisk all the ingredients in a bowl without cherries.
2. Mash the cherries in another bowl using a bowl.
3. Transfer the mashed cherries and their juices to the chocolate mixture.
4. Mix well and divide the mixture into silicone molds.
5. Freeze for 30 minutes.
6. Serve.

(29) MCT Chocolate Fat Bombs

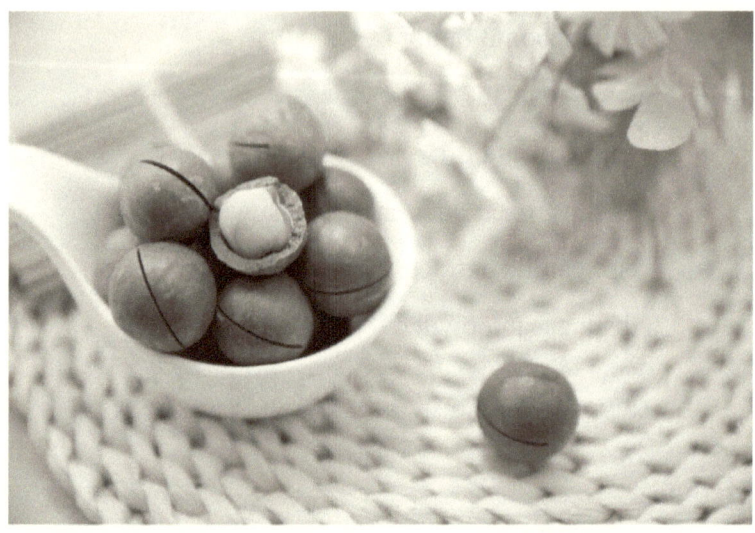

These choc0late fat bombs are no ordinary energy bites; they are loaded with macadamia nuts. The cocoa powder mix is flavored using vanilla extracts and mct oil. Serve as an after meal dessert and enjoy.

Prep Time: 10minutes

Cook Time: 0 minutes

Yield: 12

List of Ingredients:

- 4 cups macadamia nuts
- 4 tbsp. coconut oil
- 4 tbsp. MCT oil
- 2 tsp. vanilla extract
- 2/3 cup powdered sugar
- ½ cup cocoa powder

MMMMMMMMMMMMMMMMMMMMMMMMMMMMMMMMMM

Methods:

1. Grind the macadamia nuts in the food processor.
2. Add coconut oil, MCT oil, and vanilla. Blend well to puree the mixture.
3. Stir in sweetener and cocoa powder. Mix well to combine.
4. Line a muffin tray with liner and divide the mixture into the muffin cups.
5. Freeze for 30 minutes.
6. Serve.

(30) Coco Walnut Fat Bomb

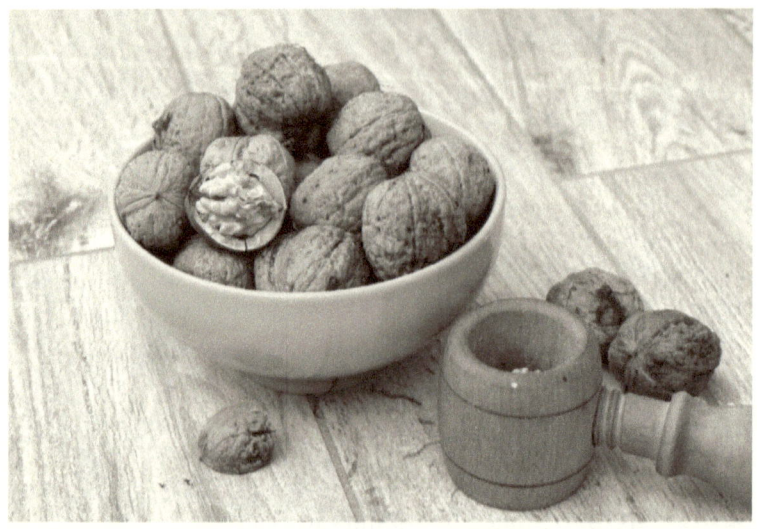

Walnuts are best for health and mind. These are nourishing for the growing children as they help strengthen the brain. Add walnuts to the simple chocolate fat bombs and make them extra delicious and super nutritious for you and your family.

Yield: 12

Prep Time: 10minutes

Cook Time: 0 minutes

List of Ingredients:

- 7 oz. dark chocolate
- ½ cup coconut oil
- 2/3 cup small walnut pieces
- 2 tsp. cinnamon
- Honey, to taste

MMMMMMMMMMMMMMMMMMMMMMMMMMMMMMMMMMM

Methods:

1. Melt chocolate and coconut oil by heating a microwave for 30 seconds.
2. Finely crush the walnuts in the food processor and transfer it to a plate.
3. Mix crushed walnuts with honey, cinnamon and chocolate mixture.
4. Divide this mixture into silicone molds.
5. Freeze for 5 minutes.
6. Top each bomb with a walnut piece.
7. Freeze for 20 minutes.
8. Serve.

(31) Buttery Cinnamon Fat Bombs

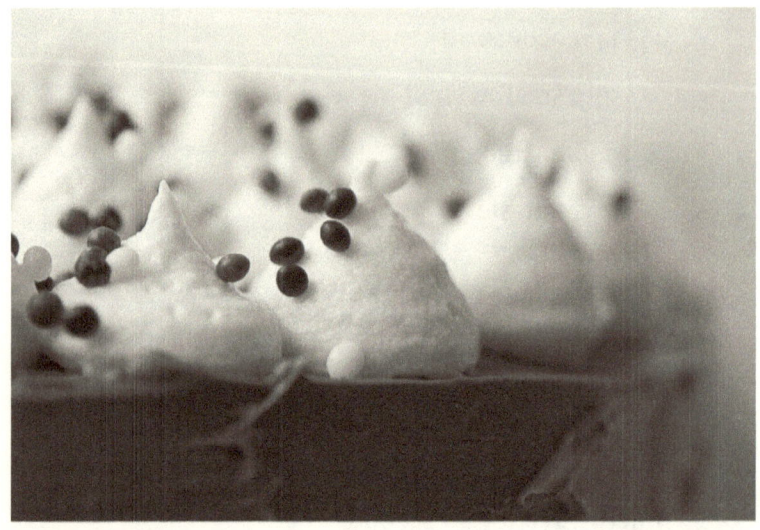

These fat bombs are all butter. Cinnamon along with vanilla sparks a balance yet distinctive flavor. These bombs can be stored easily for a longer duration, as long as you keep them in a sealed jar. Keep them in a cool place to preserve their form and taste.

Yield: 12

Prep Time: 10minutes

Cook Time: 0 minutes

List of Ingredients:

- 2 pounds salted butter, preferably grass-fed
- Honey, to taste
- 2 tbsp. cinnamon
- 3 tsp. vanilla extract
- Salt to taste, if using unsalted butter

MMMMMMMMMMMMMMMMMMMMMMMMMMMMMMMMMM

Methods:

1. Blend butter with honey, vanilla extract, and cinnamon in a food processor.
2. Divide this mixture into the silicone molds
3. Refrigerate for 1 hour.
4. Serve.

About the Author

A native of Indianapolis, Indiana, Valeria Ray found her passion for cooking while she was studying English Literature at Oakland City University. She decided to try a cooking course with her friends and the experience changed her forever. She enrolled at the Art Institute of Indiana which offered extensive courses in the culinary Arts. Once Ray dipped her toe in the cooking world, she never looked back.

When Valeria graduated, she worked in French restaurants in the Indianapolis area until she became the head chef at one of the 5-star establishments in the area. Valeria's attention to taste and visual detail caught the eye of a local business person who expressed an interest in publishing her recipes. Valeria began her secondary career authoring cookbooks and e-books which she tackled with as much talent and gusto as her first career. Her passion for food leaps off the page of her books which have colourful anecdotes and stunning pictures of dishes she has prepared herself.

Valeria Ray lives in Indianapolis with her husband of 15 years, Tom, her daughter, Isobel and their loveable Golden Retriever, Goldy. Valeria enjoys cooking special dishes in her large, comfortable kitchen where the family gets involved in preparing meals. This successful, dynamic chef is an inspiration to culinary students and novice cooks everywhere.

••••••••• ● ● ● ● ● ● •••••••

Author's Afterthoughts

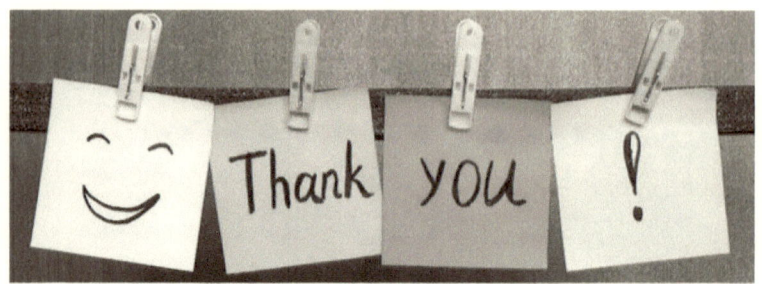

Thank you for Purchasing my book and taking the time to read it from front to back. I am always grateful when a reader chooses my work and I hope you enjoyed it!

With the vast selection available online, I am touched that you chose to be purchasing my work and take valuable time out of your life to read it. My hope is that you feel you made the right decision.

I very much would like to know what you thought of the book. Please take the time to write an honest and informative review on Amazon.com. Your experience and opinions will be of great benefit to me and those readers looking to make an informed choice.

With much thanks,

Valeria Ray

www.ingramcontent.com/pod-product-compliance
Lightning Source LLC
Chambersburg PA
CBHW021239280526
45784CB00005B/2159